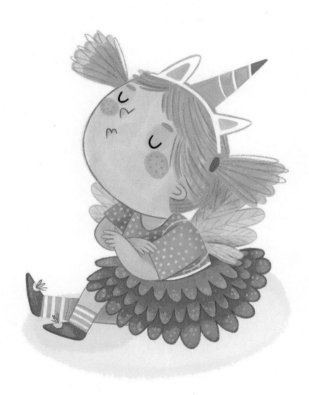

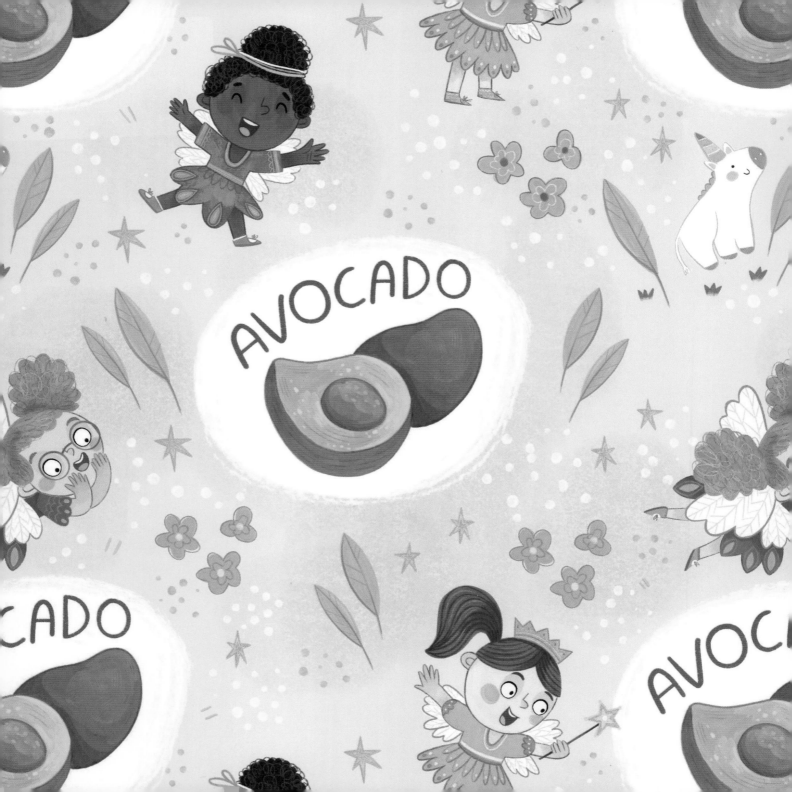

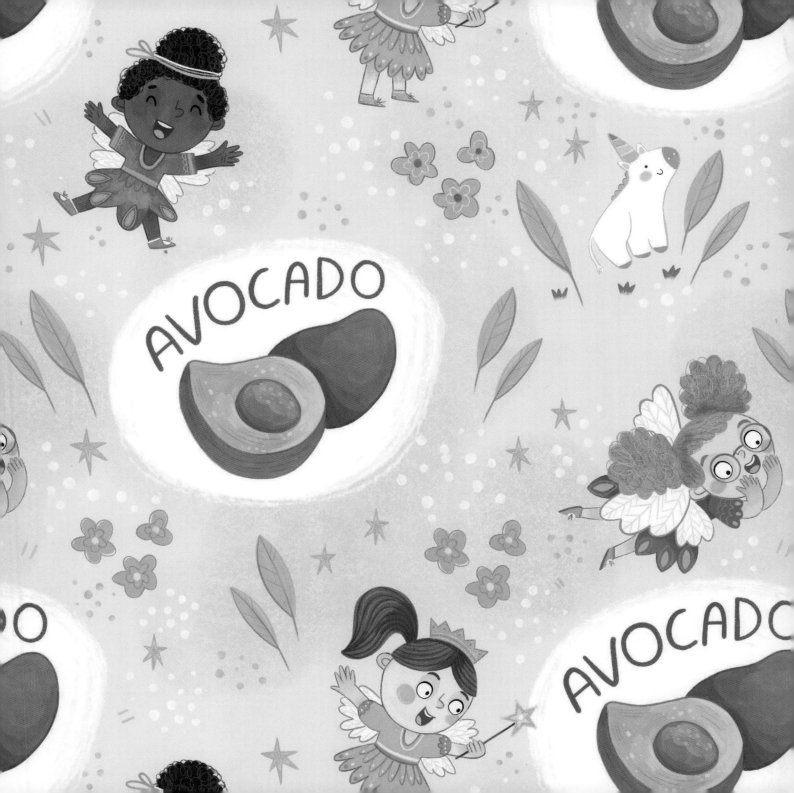

I will NEVER EVER eaT avocado

written by
ANA BALL

illustrated by
ANASTASIIA BIELIK

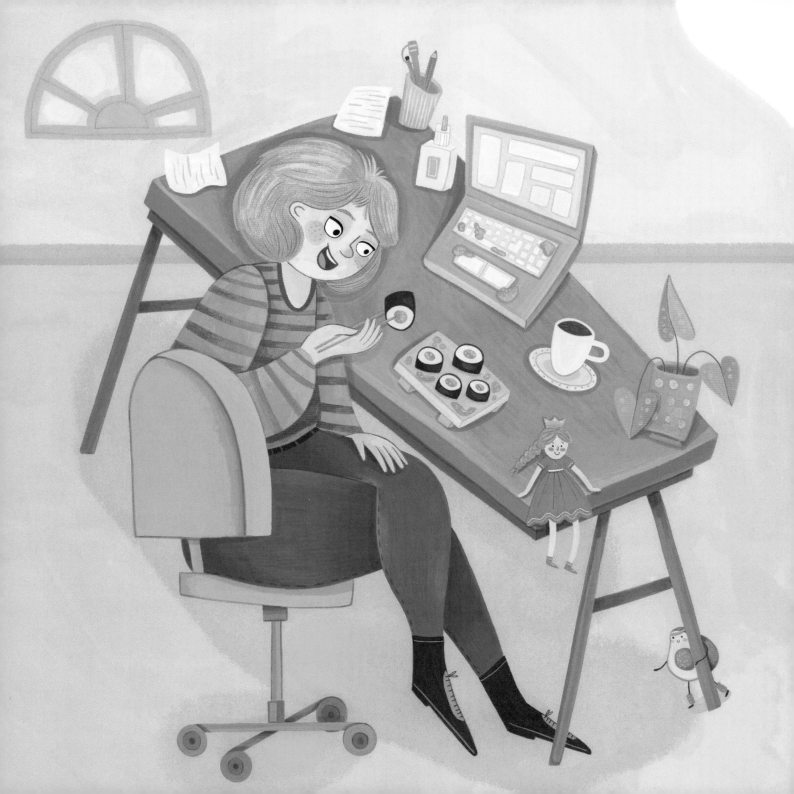

Mummy Loves
AVOCADO
- it's all over her computer

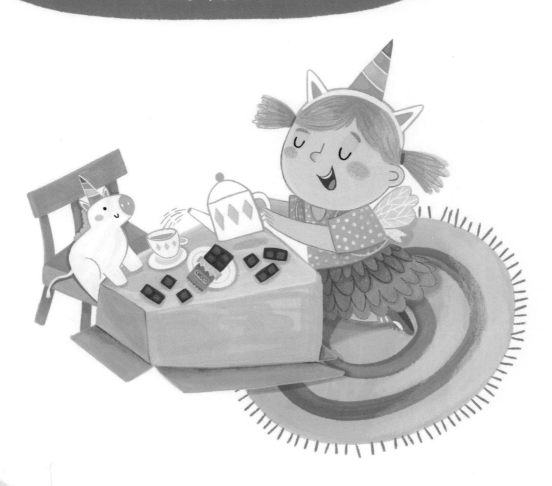

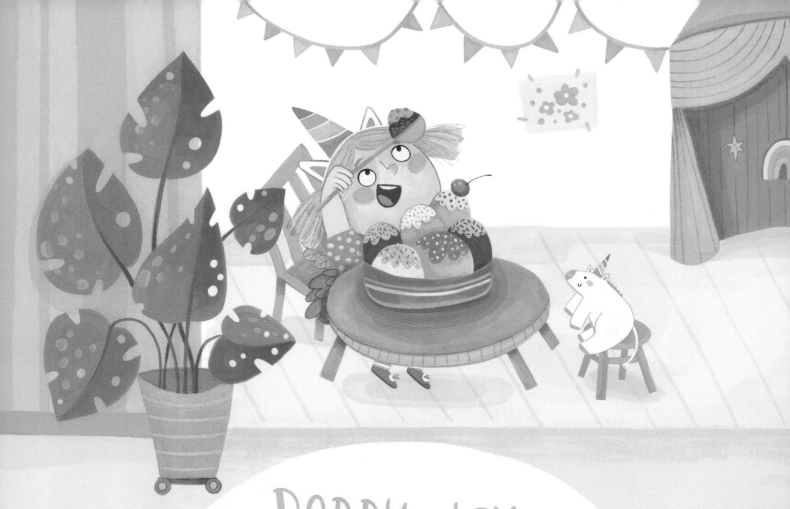

DADDY LOVES

AVOCADO

-it's all over his newspaper

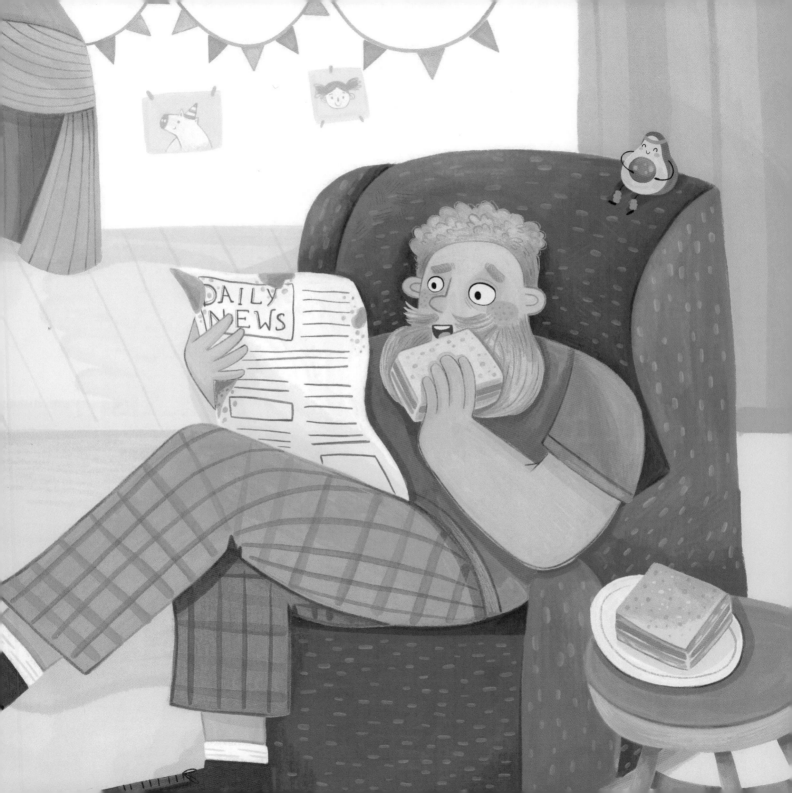

And even my baby sister Loves **AVOCADO**

-it's all over her face

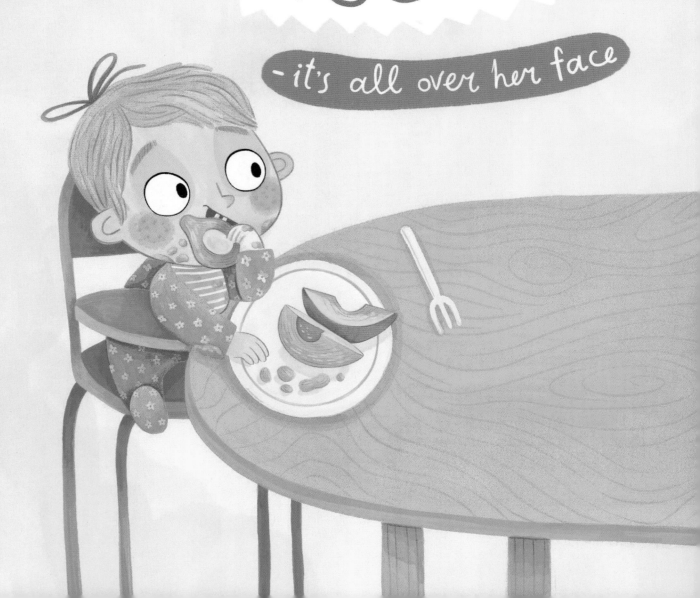

BUT I will NEVER EVER eat avocado!

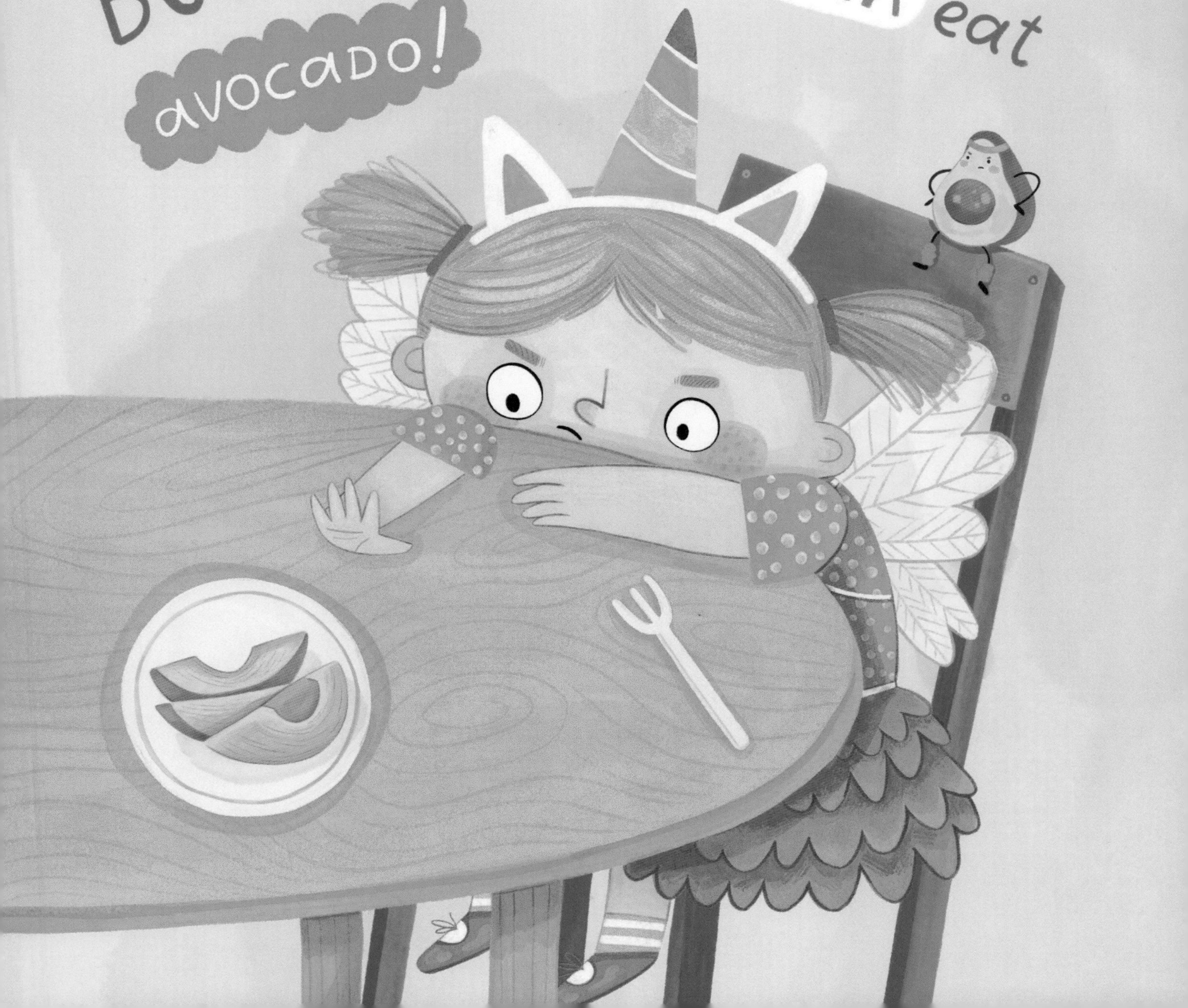

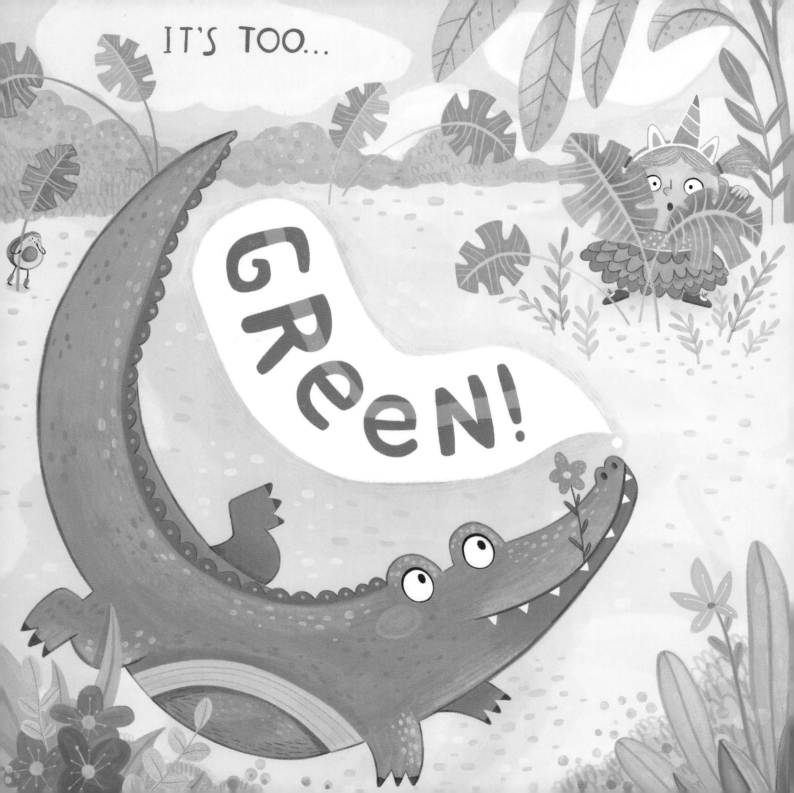

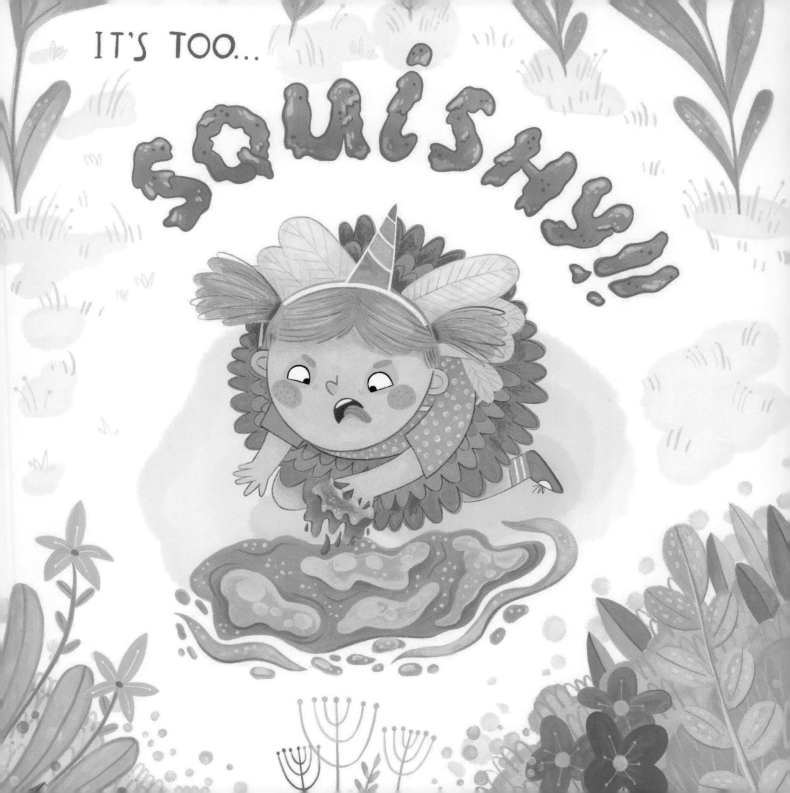

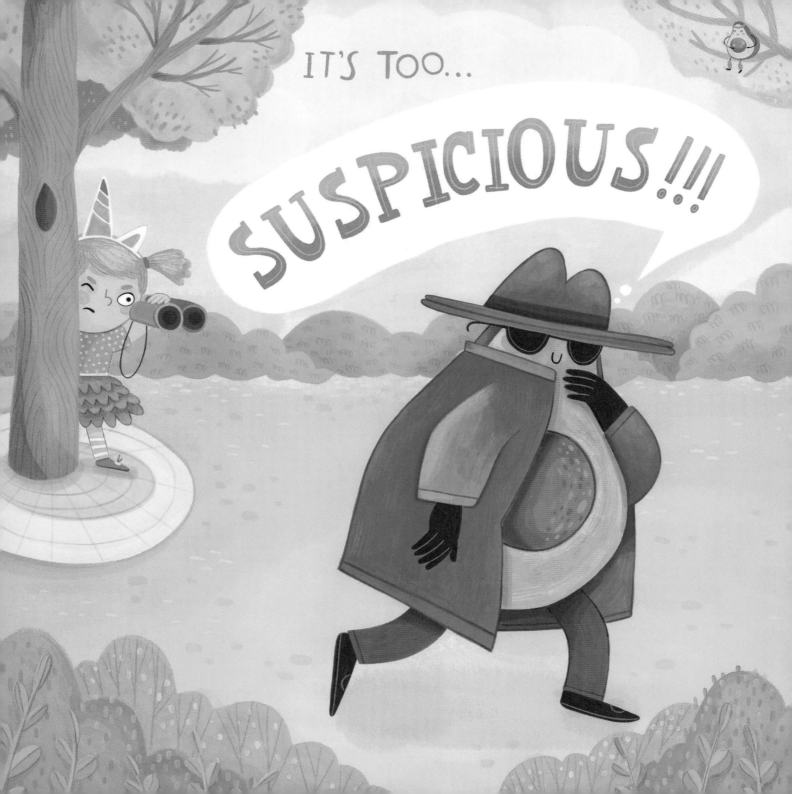

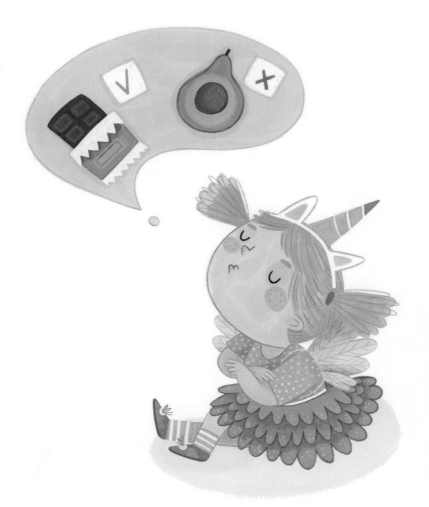

AND IT'S NOT

CHOCOLATY

ENOUGH!!!!!

My BIG sister says she DOES NOT LIKE AVOCADO either, but she LOVES that extremely chocolaty MILKSHAKE.

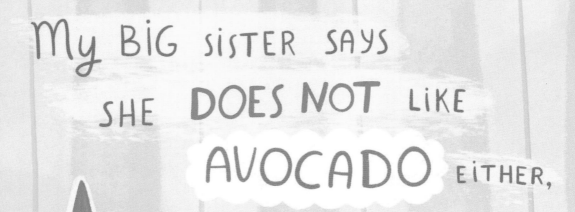
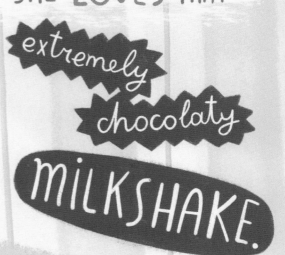

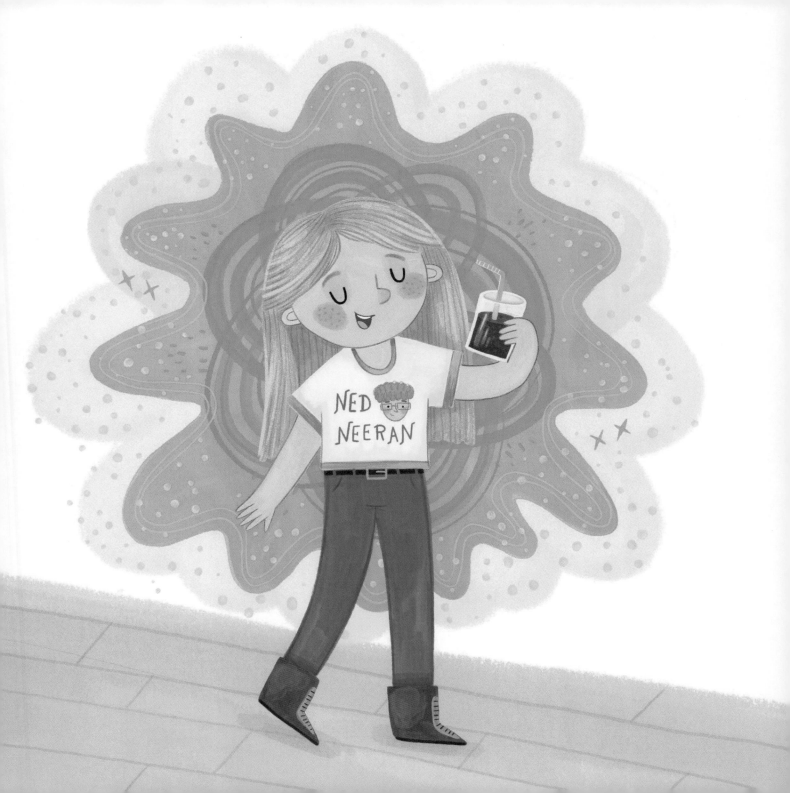

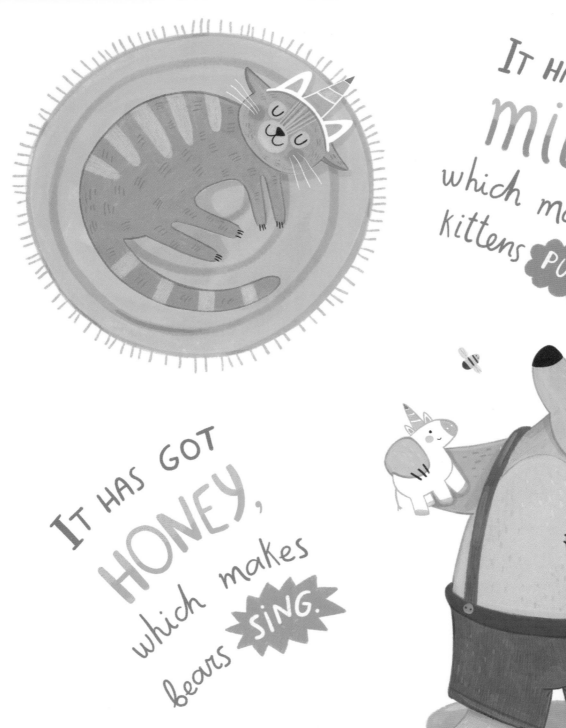

IT HAS GOT **MILK,** which makes kittens **PURR.**

IT HAS GOT **HONEY,** which makes bears **SING.**

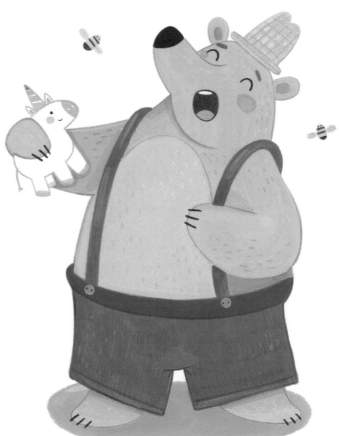

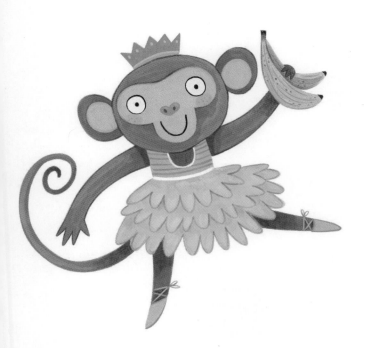

IT HAS GOT **BANANAS**, which makes monkeys **JUMP**.

IT HAS GOT **CHOCOLATE**, which makes your tummy **SMILE**.

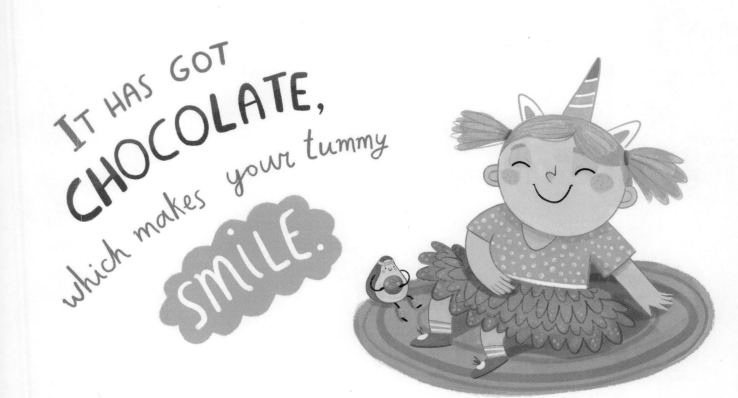

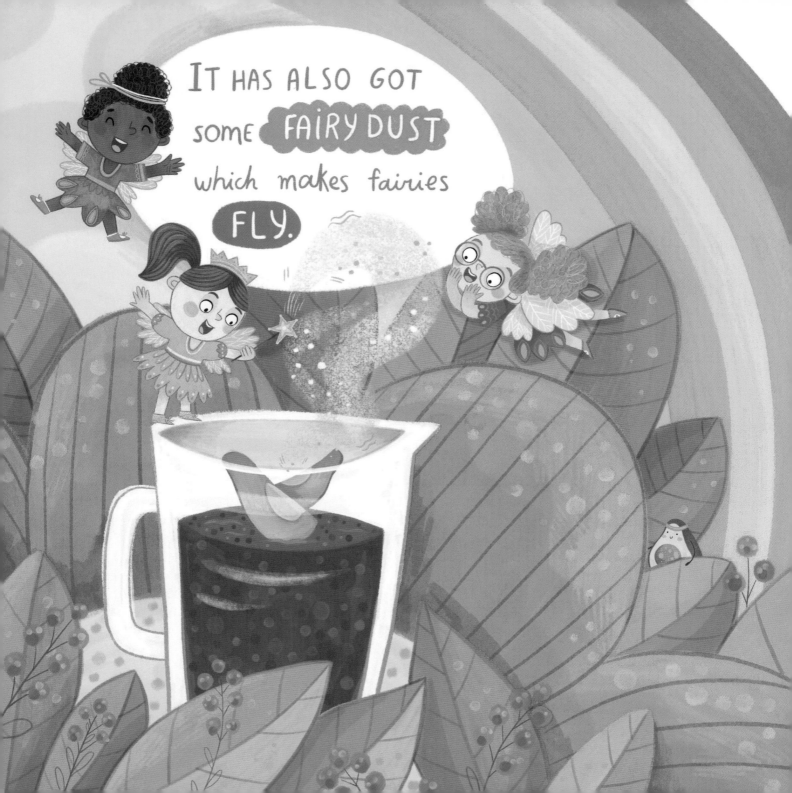

AND it's super-duper

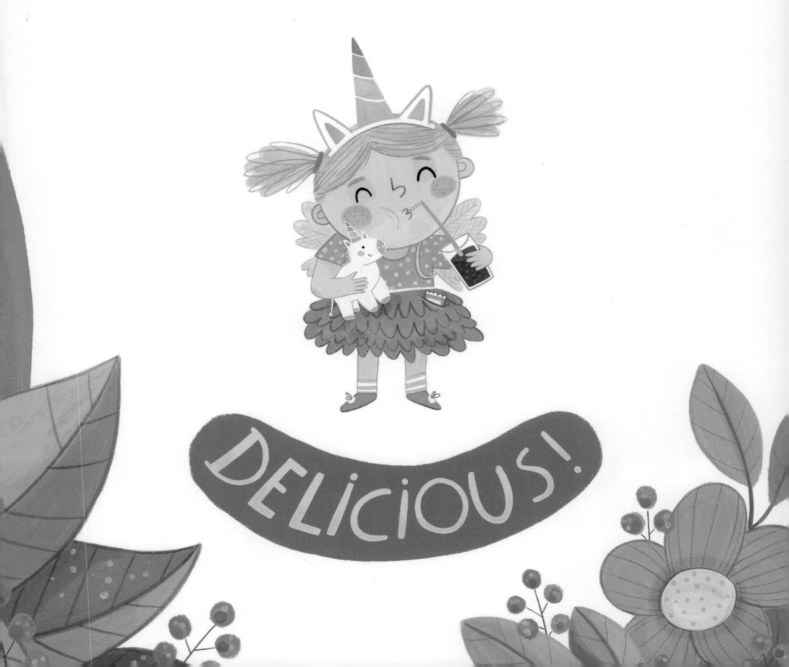

DELICIOUS!

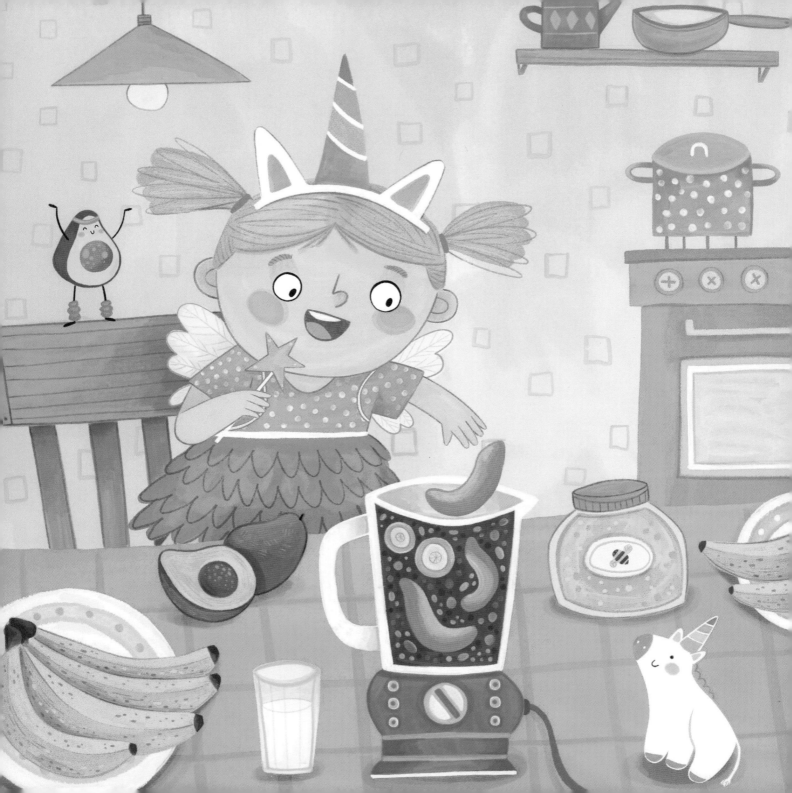

EXTREMELY CHOCOLATY milkshake Recipe

(INGREDIENTS FOR 2 small Tummies)

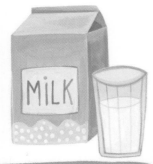
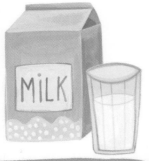

- ONE CUP OF MILK
  (CAN BE REPLACED WITH THE TASTIEST ALMOND OR COCONUT ALTERNATIVE)

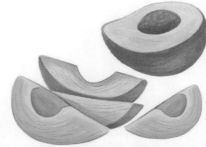

- ONE QUARTER OF a MEDIUM AVOCADO, PITTED AND PEELED

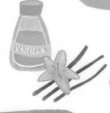

- ONE DROP OF VANILLA EXTRACT (OPTIONAL)

- ONE TEASPOON OF RUNNY HONEY

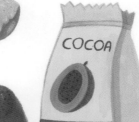

- HALF a TABLESPOON of RAW COCOA POWDER

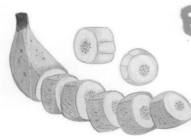

- HALF a RIPE BANANA CHOPPED (CAN BE FROZEN)

METHOD:

1. COMBINE all INGREDIENTS IN a BLENDER AND BLEND UNTIL SMOOTH.

2. TRANSFER THE MIXTURE INTO a PLASTIC CUP AND ADD a STRAW.

3. WAVE a FAIRY WAND.

4. ENJOY your DRINK!

My very VERY STRAWBERRY smoothie

(INGREDIENTS FOR 2 SMALL TUMMIES)

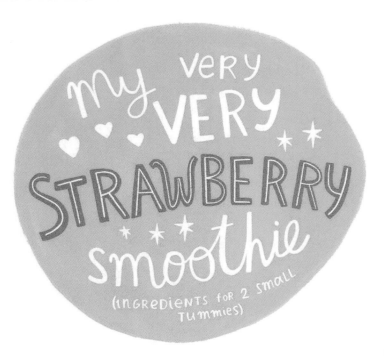

- five RASPBERRIES
- five STRAWBERRIES (CHOPPED)
- QUARTER of a BANANA
- ONE cup of MILK (CAN BE REPLACED with NON-DAIRY ALTERNATIVES)
- ONE QUARTER of a small AVOCADO (PITTED AND CHOPPED)

MILK MILK

METHOD:

1. COMBINE ALL the INGREDIENTS IN A BLENDER AND BLEND UNTIL SMOOTH.
2. TRANSFER the MIXTURE INTO TWO PLASTIC CUPS AND ADD STRAWS.
3. ENJOY!

Tip: the banana and berries can be added from frozen.

Little fish Sandwich

(Ingredients for 1 small tummy)

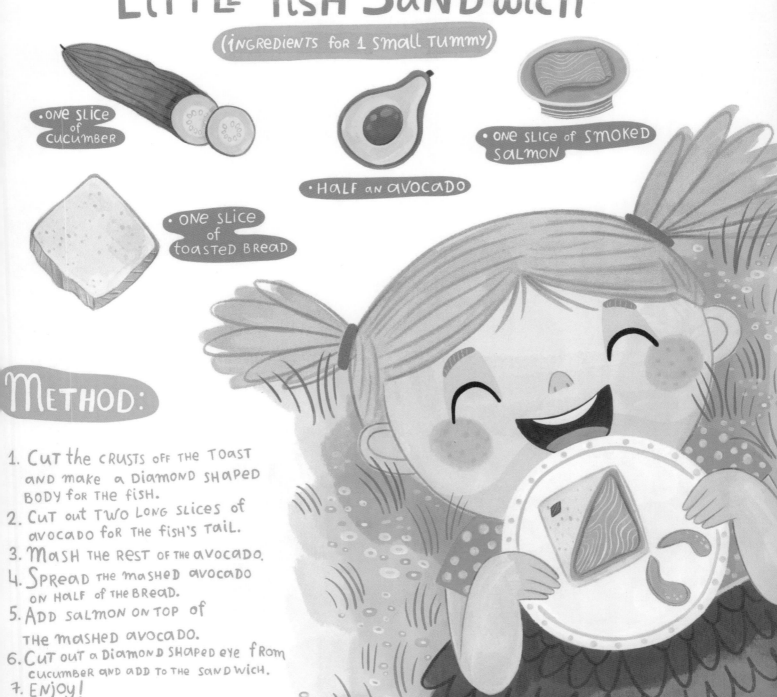

- One slice of cucumber
- Half an avocado
- One slice of smoked salmon
- One slice of toasted bread

Method:

1. Cut the crusts off the toast and make a diamond shaped body for the fish.
2. Cut out two long slices of avocado for the fish's tail.
3. Mash the rest of the avocado.
4. Spread the mashed avocado on half of the bread.
5. Add salmon on top of the mashed avocado.
6. Cut out a diamond shaped eye from cucumber and add to the sandwich.
7. Enjoy!

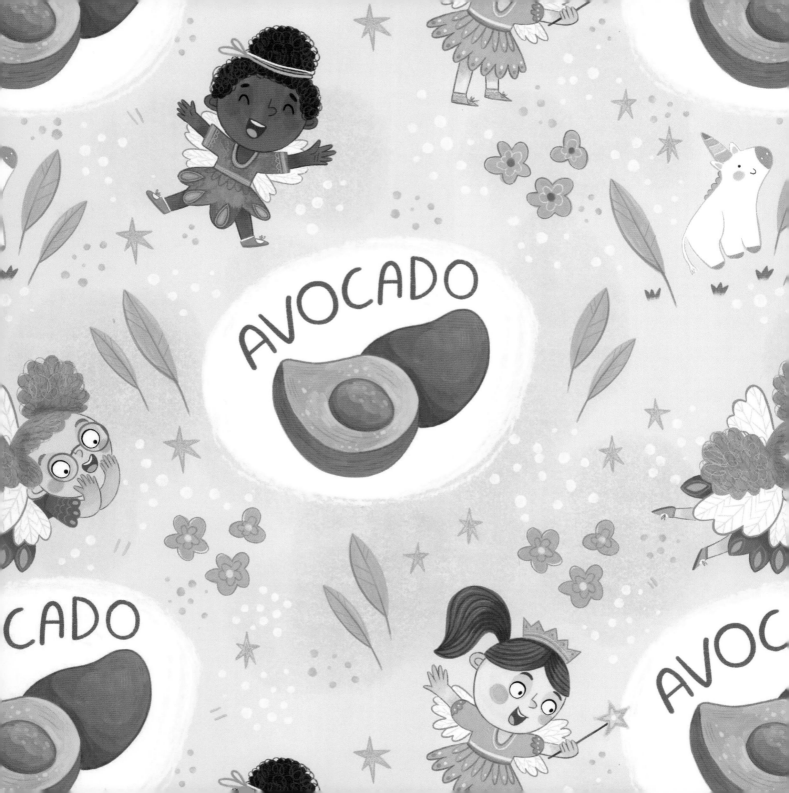

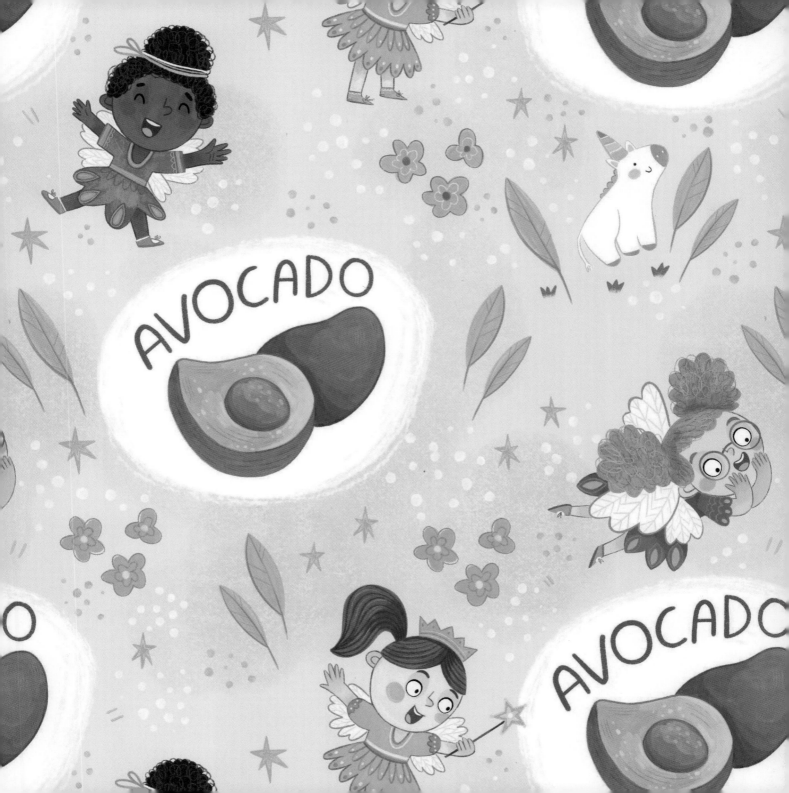

Printed in Great Britain
by Amazon

27177184R00016